When I wrote the book "Medicare is not one-size-fits-all" in June of 2013, my objective was to present a fairly neutral explanation of the different types of Medicare plans available.

I wanted people already on Medicare or getting ready to go on Medicare to understand that different Medicare plans are right for different people. I had met too many people who were in the wrong Medicare plan for their needs simply because they assumed the plan chosen by their neighbor or friend or even the only plan sold by the first Medicare insurance agent to contact them was as good as any other.

Once, I even met a realtor who had chosen a Medicare Advantage plan because the homeowner for whom she wanted sell a house worked for that company and sold only that plan. This realtor had a health condition that required her to pay thousands of dollars a year in out-of-pocket costs for which she would have had to pay nothing with a Medicare Supplement. She ended up not selling the house and will pay thousands of dollars she could have avoided with a Medicare Supplement the rest of her life.

I saw this thinking cost many people a lot of money when they became sick and, even worse, jeopardize or limit their access to the health care they deserved when they needed it most.

The response to "Medicare is not one-size-fits-all" has been overwhelming and humbling. Many people have told me my book was the only information on Medicare they could find that actually explained their options in language they could understand.

I am proud that there are many people today who have chosen Medicare plans that are right for them both now and in the future because they read my book and better understood their choices.
While my book "Medicare is not one-size-fits-all" is a fairly neutral explanation of Medicare options, I am not neutral about which type of Medicare plans are best for most people.

I believe almost all Medicare beneficiaries should stay on Original Medicare and have a Medicare Supplement and a Medicare Part D Drug Plan.

This approach gives the Medicare beneficiary the best chance for a good health outcome when they become sick. This approach also eliminates the potential for unexpected health conditions to lead to tens of thousands of dollars in unexpected out-of-pocket costs that can jeopardize a retiree's finances.

A close friend of mine is the leading Primary Care Physician in a mid-sized town in Texas. A few months ago she told me the following:

> *"The best health outcomes I have with my patients are those with the Original Red, White and Blue Medicare Card and a Medicare Supplement Card such as Mutual of Omaha. I am able to get them the treatment they need and I can get them into whatever specialists are right for them. I am not always able to do that with my patients who have Medicare Advantage plans and sometimes that leads to worse health outcomes."*

> *Primary Care Physician*

After assisting more than a thousand Medicare beneficiaries choose a Medicare insurance plan and hearing the stories of when they had previously chosen a wrong Medicare plan, my core belief about selecting a Medicare insurance plan is as follows:

Choosing a Medicare plan is not about selecting a plan that will cost you the least money when you are healthy. Choosing a Medicare plan is about selecting a plan that will provide the maximum access to the health care you need and deserve with little or no unexpected costs when you are sick so you have the best chance of having the best health outcome possible.

On the following pages are the Top Ten reasons I recommend Original Medicare combined with a Medicare Supplement and a stand-alone Medicare Part D Drug Plan instead of a privately administered Medicare Advantage plan.

Top Ten Reasons I recommend Medicare Supplements

1) Original Medicare is more likely to approve a surgery or treatment your doctor believes is right for you than a Medicare Advantage plan.

With a Medicare Advantage plan, someone other than you and your doctor is in a position to decide whether to spend the money on the surgery or treatment your doctor chooses.

Your health care decisions should be between you and your doctor. A budget analyst sitting in a cubicle with a spreadsheet evaluating the cost versus benefit of the treatment your doctor believes is right for you should not have a decision-making role in your health care.

2) **With Original Medicare you have the maximum choice and ability to see specialists and providers who are best for your unique health situation. With a Medicare Advantage plan, you are limited to specialists and providers in their network.**

A couple of years ago I received a call from a lady in Houston whose husband had just been diagnosed with life-threatening cancer. Her husband had gone on Medicare only two months before and had been talked into enrolling in a Medicare Advantage plan by a salesman who stressed how he would receive a free health club membership and $100 worth of eyeglasses every year if he withdrew from Original Medicare and enrolled in the Medicare Advantage plan he was selling.

This couple only lived a few miles from M.D. Anderson Cancer Center which is regarded as one of the premier cancer treatment facilities in the world. However, his new Medicare Advantage plan excluded his receiving cancer treatment from M.D. Anderson.

Because this gentleman was still within his first six months on Medicare, I was able to enroll him in a Medicare Supplement so he could return to Original Medicare and receive care from the world-renowned doctors at M.D. Anderson. As a bonus, he paid nothing out-of-pocket for his treatment beyond the monthly premium for his Medicare Supplement whereas he would have paid thousands of dollars under his former Medicare Advantage plan.

3) **Being in a Medicare Advantage plan can result in unexpected expenses of tens of thousands of dollars if one becomes seriously and/or chronically ill.**

Many chronic health conditions such as cancer, diabetes, COPD and even arthritis and macular degeneration require continual and permanent treatments that cost Medicare Advantage members thousands of dollars year after year. Anyone who is enrolled in a Medicare Advantage plan is vulnerable to numerous common health conditions that could wreak havoc on their finances the rest of their life.

4) Because Medicare Supplements require health underwriting for anyone who has been on Medicare more than 6 months, someone enrolled in a Medicare Advantage plan who is suddenly required to pay thousands of dollars in unexpected costs because they are sick and need treatment will likely find themselves ineligible for a Medicare Supplement due to their health condition.

The only time someone can be certain of being approved for a Medicare Supplement is when they first go on Medicare Part B - usually when they turn 65. Once someone has been on Medicare Part B more than 6 months and has developed a serious health condition, they are likely to be turned down for a Medicare Supplement even though that is the time they need a Medicare Supplement the most.

5) **People who take expensive medications can often get them at a lower overall cost with a stand-alone Medicare Part D Drug Plan that with a Medicare Part D Drug Plan included in a Medicare Advantage plan.**

Medicare beneficiaries in most states can choose among at least 30 or 40 stand-alone Medicare Part D Drug Plans. On the other hand, there are often as few as three or four Part D Drug Plans available with Medicare Advantage plans.

This greater choice makes it likely someone can find a stand-alone drug plan more tailored to their specific mix of medications and, therefore, at a lower overall cost. I have had clients who were able to save more than $1,000 a year on their medications by choosing a stand-alone Medicare Part D drug plan instead of getting their medications through a Medicare Advantage plan.

6) **Medicare Advantage plans can and will change significantly over time in terms of which doctors are in their networks, how much a member must pay when they become sick, what medications they cover and when they approve specific treatments.**

However, even though a Medicare Advantage plan may change significantly and become much less of a good fit and value for the member, the member's health may still prevent them from changing to a Medicare Supplement.

7) **If your doctor leaves a Medicare Advantage plan, you will likely be forced to change doctors.**

I have seen situations in which a Medicare Advantage plan terminated a large group of doctors during the middle of the year and forced all of its members who used those doctors to find a new doctor. I once met a Medicare Advantage member who was scheduled for cancer surgery the first day of a month and his surgeon was terminated from his Medicare Advantage plan at the end of the previous month. This cancer patient was forced to delay his surgery and find a new surgeon who was unfamiliar with his situation.

8) I have never had someone with Original Medicare and a Medicare Supplement who had a health problem tell me they wished they had a Medicare Advantage plan in which they had to pay thousands of dollars in unexpected costs when they became sick. I have met many Medicare Advantage members who were sick express regret and dismay that they were in a plan that was costing them thousands of dollars and, even worse, limiting their access to the health care they needed.

Unfortunately, most of these Medicare Advantage members who were paying thousands of dollars in unexpected costs told me they did not understand when they enrolled in a Medicare Advantage plan that they would be locked into this type of plan the rest of their lives if they had a health condition that would cause them to be declined for a Medicare Supplement after they had been on Medicare more than six months.

9) If you have a health condition and you want to make sure you see the best doctors possible for your condition, you can likely see those doctors with a Medicare Supplement and not have to pay any out-of-pocket costs. This is true even if those doctors are in another state or even across the country. With a Medicare Advantage plan, you can only see the doctors in your plan's network which are usually doctors close to where you live.

If my son or daughter was diagnosed with a type of cancer that I did not believe the doctors where I lived had sufficient expertise and experience in successfully treating and there was a doctor somewhere else who had such expertise and experience, then I would take my son or daughter to that doctor.

Someone with Original Medicare combined with a Medicare Supplement can do just that to give themselves the best chance for the best health outcome possible.

With a Medicare Advantage-type plan, that same person would have limited choices in doctors and would in all likelihood not be able to see the doctor he or she felt could provide the best treatment. Ironically, they would likely have to pay thousands of dollars in unexpected costs for treatment from a doctor or hospital they did not want to use in the first place.

10) **The Affordable Care Act is cutting the funding for Medicare Advantage plans and will likely continue to do do.**

I try not to take sides politically when helping people with Medicare. However, for the past three years the federal government, as part of the Affordable Care Act, has reduced funding for Medicare Advantage plans resulting in more limited networks of doctors, less approvals for treatments, less coverage for drugs and higher out-of-pocket costs paid by members for medical services and medications.

In today's political climate, being locked into a Medicare Advantage is not the best place to be in terms of controlling costs and maximizing access to health care.

Bonus Section

How Medicare Works in Plain English

How Medicare Works

What Medicare Covers

Medicare covers most health care services - hospital stays, surgeries, doctor visits, tests, home health care, medications, rehabilitation and many more.

Medicare generally does not cover such services as dental care, cosmetic services, routine vision, hearing and long-term custodial care due to chronic conditions or cognitive impairment.

When you are on Medicare you can generally go to any doctor or medical facility that takes Medicare at any location throughout the United States. You do not need referrals to see specialists and you do not have to choose a Primary Care Doctor.

Medicare has three parts - Part A, Part B and Part D. Part A and Part B have been the primary parts of Medicare since it was created by Congress in 1965. Part D drug plans were added by Congress in 2006.

Medicare Part A

Medicare Part A consists of the costs of going into a hospital as an in-patient, the costs of facility-based skilled nursing care and the costs of three pints of blood. There is no monthly premium for Part A and one becomes automatically eligible for Part A the first day of the month in which they turn 65 providing they or their spouse have worked the minimum time and paid accordingly into the Medicare system during their working lives.

The costs the Medicare beneficiary must pay under Medicare Part A are substantial. When one goes into the hospital as an in-patient, the deductible is $1,216. What this means is a one-night hospital stay can result in a bill for the Medicare member of $1,184. For skilled nursing care, after 20 days the Medicare member pays $152 per day. A Medicare beneficiary in a skilled nursing facility for the full 100 days for which Medicare will pay would be responsible for paying $12,160.

Since Medicare generally requires a skilled nursing stay be preceded by a hospital stay, a Medicare member who goes into the hospital for a period of time and then spends the maximum 100 days in a skilled nursing facility would be responsible for a total bill of $13,376.

Medicare Part B

Medicare Part B consists of all other Medicare-covered services such as doctor visits, outpatient services, x-rays, lab work, home health care, preventive screenings and Part B medications which are medications administered in a medical facility such as a doctor's office or hospital.

With Part B, there is a premium which in 2014 is $104.90 per month. For people who collect Social Security, the monthly premium is deducted from their monthly Social Security check.

Just like Part A, one becomes eligible for Part B the first day of the month in which they turn 65. However, people who choose to continue their insurance through an employer may choose not to take Part B when they first turn 65. Someone who chooses to defer Part B due to continuing employer coverage will be able to select it once they leave the employer coverage in the future.

Part B has an annual deductible of $147. After this $147 deductible is reached, Medicare plays 80 percent of Part B expenses while the Medicare beneficiary is responsible for the remaining 20 percent.

While a 20 percent cost share may not seem substantial, in reality it can result in large bills for the Medicare beneficiary. For example, if someone had cancer and had a sizable amount of chemotherapy, the costs can easily add up to tens of thousands of dollars of which 20 percent would be a large amount.

Very importantly, there is no out-of-pocket maximum with Medicare as there is with many other types of health insurance.

Medicare Part D

Medicare Part D consists of drug coverage in which Medicare beneficiaries pay co-pays rather than the full costs of medications. Part D plans have monthly premiums and can either be purchased as a stand-alone plan or can be included in a Medicare Advantage plan. Medicare beneficiaries are eligible to enroll in a Part D plan once they become eligible for Part A.

Summary

Medicare covers most, though not all, of the type of medical services Medicare beneficiaries may need. However, it does not cover these services with little or not cost to the beneficiary.

Most Medicare beneficiaries will need some type of additional Medicare insurance coverage to protect them from substantial and unexpected costs. The remainder of this book will focus on these types of plans and how the Medicare beneficiary can evaluate what type of plan is right for them as well as which specific plan is best for them.

Covering Your Medicare Costs

Medicare Insurance Plans

As we just discussed, while Medicare covers most health-related services and pays a majority of the cost, the Medicare beneficiary is still responsible for a substantial portion that can be very large with certain medical conditions and treatments. Most Medicare beneficiaries choose to enroll in an additional Medicare insurance plan rather than risk huge, unlimited and unexpected bills.

There are two primary types of Medicare insurance plans that limit the financial exposure of Medicare beneficiaries while still providing access to the Medicare benefits they may need. The first type is a traditional Medicare Supplement. A Medicare Supplement is a simple plan. In return for the Medicare beneficiary paying a monthly premium, a private insurance carrier assumes the financial responsibility for all or part of the Medicare beneficiary's share of Medicare costs.

With a Medicare Supplement, the Medicare beneficiary essentially locks in his or her costs so these costs will not fluctuate regardless of the type of health year they experience. For example, with a Medicare supplement the Medicare beneficiary would incur no more medical costs during a year in which they may have been hospitalized numerous times than a year in which they had no health issues at all and only visited their doctors for an annual checkup.

While many Medicare beneficiaries choose the Medicare Supplement approach to managing their Medicare costs, others choose a relatively new type of plan called Medicare Advantage.

Medicare Advantage plans work almost exactly the opposite of the way Medicare Supplements work. With a Medicare Advantage plan, a Medicare beneficiary pays little or no monthly premium but instead pays co-pays and co-insurance as they receive medical care. Unlike regular Medicare, there is an out-of-pocket maximum for what the beneficiary can pay in total co-pays and co-insurance. In addition, many Medicare Advantage plans provide additional benefits beyond those provided by regular Medicare and Medicare Supplements.

How do Medicare Supplements Work?

Medicare Supplements are the simplest type of Medicare insurance. Medicare Supplements pay all or part of the Medicare beneficiary's share of Medicare costs.

When a Medicare beneficiary has a Medicare Supplement, they provide both their government-issued Medicare card as well as the carrier-provided Medicare Supplement card whenever they receive medical services. The provider then bills Medicare for its share and the Medicare Supplement carrier for its share.

Medicare Supplement Plan Types

There are different versions of Medicare Supplements that are standardized across the various insurance carriers that offer them. For example, Plan F pays all co-pays, co-insurance and deductibles so that the Medicare beneficiary never pays anything out of pocket for Medicare-covered services other than the monthly premium.

Very importantly, Plan F provides the same coverage regardless of which insurance carrier provides it.

Another Medicare Supplement version - Plan G - pays all costs except for the annual Part B deductible of $147. However, the annual premiums for Plan G are often several hundred dollars less than the comparable premium for Plan F. By selecting Plan G, the Medicare beneficiary can often save substantial money over the course of the full year.

Another Medicare Supplement plan - Plan N - requires Medicare beneficiaries to pay a $20 co-pay when visiting the doctor. However, as with Plan G, the additional out-of-pocket costs is usually outweighed by the savings in monthly premiums over the full year.

Medicare Supplement Rates

Medicare Supplement rates are based on a number of factors including:

1. Age
2. Gender
3. Location
4. Tobacco use
5. Discounts for married couples
6. Payment frequency and method

Very importantly, Medicare Supplement rates can and likely will increase over times based on three different factors:

1. The increasing age of the Medicare beneficiary
2. The overall claims experience of all people in the plan
3. Inflation in the health care economy

When evaluating a Medicare Supplement, it is important to examine not only the current rates at age 65 or whatever age at which Medicare beneficiary is considering enrollment but also to review the rate at which the rates increase with age.

Some carriers have lower rates at age 65 than other carriers but more than make up for it with higher age-based increases in the future. At any time, a prospective Medicare Supplement enrollee can review not only the rates for his or her age but the rates for all ages.

Medicare Supplement Underwriting

Medicare Supplements are underwritten based on the enrollee's health. This means when one applies for a Medicare Supplement, they are required to disclose any pre-existing health conditions they may have. Having conditions such as insulin-dependent diabetes, heart problems or obesity will likely cause someone to be declined for coverage.

There is one major exception to this underwriting. When someone is first going on Medicare Part B - usually at age 65 - they have a 6-month window in which to enroll in any Medicare Supplement without being asked any health questions.

This means that someone with chronic health problems who could greatly benefit from the "no out-of-pocket costs" structure of a Medicare Supplement can get this coverage only at this point in his or her life. Importantly, once they are enrolled in a Medicare Supplement they can continue the coverage the rest of their life as long as they pay their premiums.

This also means that someone who may be in good health when first going on Medicare Part B but who may want such "no out-of-pocket costs" coverage in the future in case they do develop serious health problems can only be certain of being approved for such coverage when they first go on Medicare Part B.

Medicare Part D with Medicare Supplements

While there is a later chapter dedicated to Medicare Part D plans, it is important to understand that with a Medicare Supplement, it is also necessary for most Medicare beneficiaries to enroll in a separate Medicare Part D drug plan. Medicare Supplements only cover the Medicare beneficiary's share of Medicare Parts A and B.

The Medicare Part D drug plan will allow the beneficiary to pay only smaller co-pays instead of full price for any medications they use. This plan will also allow the Medicare beneficiary to meet to government's requirement for maintaining credible drug coverage and therefore avoid a late enrollment penalty in the future.

Medicare Advantage

How does Medicare Advantage work?

Medicare Advantage plans work very different than Medicare Supplements. Most Medicare Advantage plans have little or no monthly premium. However, unlike with a Medicare Supplement, the member is responsible for co-pays and co-insurance as he or she receive health care services. However, the co-pays and co-insurance are generally lower than they would be with regular Medicare.

Unlike regular Medicare, Medicare Advantage plans have out-of-pockets maximums which protect the member from unlimited costs in the event of a serious and expensive health condition. For most plans, out-of-pocket maximums tend to be anywhere from $3,400 to $7,000.

Many Medicare Advantage plans provide additional benefits not covered by regular Medicare such as dental and routine vision. Some Medicare Advantage plans even provide hearing aids, transportation to and from a doctor and health club memberships.

Most Medicare Advantage plans also include the Medicare Part D drug coverage so members are not required to pay for a separate drug plan.

In return for lower co-pays and co-insurance, out-of-pocket maximums and additional benefits, Medicare Advantage members agree to receive their routine medical care from the provider's network of doctors and hospitals. Depending on the specific Medicare Advantage plan, members may also agree to other requirements such as identifying a Primary Care Physician and getting referrals prior to seeing a specialist.

Does Medicare Advantage save money?

For most people who are in average or better health, choosing a Medicare Advantage plan will likely save them money over the course of their life. The reason for this is the cumulative cost of co-pays and co-insurance tends to be considerably less than the cumulative savings of not paying a monthly premium.

This cost savings is not guaranteed because if the member experiences costly health conditions the co-pays and co-insurance can exceed the savings from not paying a premium. Because of the structure of co-pays and co-insurance, there is less cost certainty with a Medicare Advantage plan than with a Medicare Supplement. In normal health years, members may only spend a couple of hundred dollars or even less. In years in which a member may be hospitalized or have extensive medical tests, procedures or treatment, he or she could pay much more up to the out-of-pocket maximum.

Types of Medicare Advantage plans

There are two primary types of Medicare Advantage plans: Health Maintenance Organizations (HMOs) and Preferred Provider Organizations (PPOs).

In an HMO, all health care other than emergency or urgent care must be obtained from the plan's provider network. When the member has an emergency or urgent health care need, they can receive care at any provider and it will be considered in-network.

With most HMOs, the member is usually required to designate a Primary Care Provider. With many, but not all HMOs, the member must get a referral from the Primary Care Provider prior to seeing a specialist.

In a PPO, members can choose to receive care from a non-network provider though their share of the cost will usually be higher than with an in-network provider. As with an HMO, treatment for an emergency or urgent care situation is considered in-network regardless of where it is received.

With a PPO, members usually are not required to designate a Primary Care Physician nor are they required to get referrals prior to seeing a specialist.

Supplements Or Advantage

Which one is right for me?

Medicare is not a "one-size-fits-all" product. The best plan for one person can be the wrong plan for someone else.

As this book indicates, I almost always recommend a Medicare Supplement instead of a Medicare Advantage Plan. The reasons for this are two-fold:

1) When some becomes sick, they will have much more choice and access to care with a Medicare Supplement than with a Medicare Advantage Plan. More choice and more access in health care leads to better health outcomes.

2) While the costs can be less with a Medicare Advantage plan when one is healthy, they can be much more with the same Medicare Advantage plan when one becomes sick.

Regardless of one's current health situation, I consider a Medicare Supplement an excellent investment in one's future health and finances.

The only time I recommend a Medicare Advantage plan is if someone simply cannot afford the monthly premiums of a Medicare Supplement.

The correct approach to choosing a Medicare plan is to go through a careful process that identifies one's needs and preferences and then aligns them with the plan and carrier available in their area that best meets those needs and preferences.

The following are overall guidelines for choosing between a Medicare Supplement and a Medicare Advantage plan:

Health

When someone has chronic health conditions at age 65 that require significantly higher than average health care services, one should choose a Medicare Supplement if they can afford it.

There are two reasons for this. First, when one is turning 65, they have a once-in-a-lifetime opportunity to enroll in a Medicare Supplement without having to disclose existing or past health conditions. Chronic conditions such as diabetes, COPD or Congestive Heart Failure or even past conditions such as many types of cancer can make someone ineligible for a Medicare Supplement once they are 6 months past their 65th birthday.

While someone can switch from a Medicare Supplement to a Medicare Advantage plan in the future, a person with chronic health conditions will likely be unable to switch from a Medicare Advantage plan to a Medicare Supplement.

The second reason someone with chronic health conditions should choose a Medicare Supplement is it is possible the cumulative cost of their co-pays will exceed what they would have paid during the year for a Medicare Supplement that would have paid all of their out-of-pocket expenses.

Taken together, these two reasons make it likely a Medicare Supplement is the best choice for someone with serious chronic health conditions.

Finances

If one cannot afford the monthly premiums required of a Medicare Supplement and a stand-alone Medicare Part D Drug plan, then a Medicare Advantage plan is likely the right approach.

It does not make sense for someone to pay a premium for a Medicare Supplement to avoid the costs of catastrophic health conditions and then not be able to afford their monthly medicines, groceries or utilities.

Doctors and hospitals are much more willing to work with someone to pay co-pays over time than pharmacies, grocery stores or utility companies.

Lifestyles

Someone who travels extensively out of their home area should consider a Medicare Supplement. While Medicare Advantage plans allow for members to receive emergency or urgent care outside of their provider network and have it billed as in-network, there are many types of routine care that someone may wish to receive while away from home. This is particularly true for someone who spends a large part of the year at a second home a considerable distance from their primary home.

Personal Preferences and Choices

A person who wants maximum choice and flexibility concerning their health care should probably choose a Medicare Supplement. Of course, the price for this choice and flexibility is the likely higher cumulative premiums with a Medicare Supplement than the sum of co-pays and co-insurance with a Medicare Advantage plan.

If someone wants the flexibility to go to the Mayo Clinic or Johns Hopkins or a nationally-renowned Orthopedic surgeon, a Medicare Supplement is likelier to provide that option than a Medicare Advantage plan.

While Medicare Advantage plans are committed to providing the health care needed to keep their members healthy, not all procedures and treatment require the best known physicians and hospitals in the country.

Medicare Part D Drug Plans

How Part D Drug Plans Work

Medicare Part D drug plans allow Medicare beneficiaries to purchase medications paying co-pays rather than the full of the medication. These drug plans can either be purchased as a stand-alone plan - usually by a Medicare beneficiary with a Medicare Supplement - or as part of a Medicare Advantage plan.

Medicare requires all Medicare beneficiaries to be enrolled in a Medicare Part D drug plan unless the beneficiary has alternative coverage that meets the Medicare standard coverage criteria. This criteria is often called "credible coverage."

Medicare members can have credible coverage outside of a Medicare Part D drug plan through such sources as group coverage through an employer or through Veterans' Administration (VA) drug benefits for beneficiaries with VA benefits.

Medicare Part D Late Enrollment Penalty

If a Medicare beneficiary does not choose to enroll in a Medicare Part D drug plan when first eligible and does not have credible coverage through an alternative source, Medicare will impose a Late Enrollment Penalty if they enroll in a plan in the future. This penalty will be 1 percent of the national average Medicare Part D monthly premium for every month they were eligible for coverage but did not elect coverage. This penalty is assessed for the remainder of one's life.

This means if someone enrolls in a Medicare Part D drug plan 5 years - or 60 months - after they were first eligible, they will pay a penalty equal to 60 percent of the Medicare Part D base beneficiary monthly premium. In 2013, average monthly premium for a Medicare Part D drug plan is $32.42. This means the beneficiary assessed this penalty due to not enrolling for 5 years will pay $19.45 (.01 X 60 X $32.42) for the rest of their life.

Medicare Part D Formulary

All Medicare Part D drug plans have a formulary which lists the medications that are covered under the plan as well as the tier to which they are assigned. Medications that are not included in the formulary are not covered. However, a member's doctor can request a non-covered medication be covered using a process called a Formulary Appeal.

With a Formulary Appeal, the plan will consider the request based on the individual situation of the member and the explanation provided by the doctor as to why the member needs the uncovered medication instead of a medication included in the formulary.

Medicare Part D Coverage Phases

Medicare Part D Drug plans have four distinct phases of coverage - the Deductible Phase (if applicable), the Initial Coverage Phase, the Coverage Gap (also called the Donut Hole) and the Catastrophic Phase.

Deductible Phase

Some, but not all, Medicare Part D drug plans have a deductible. The standard deductible in 2013 is $310. This means the Medicare beneficiary will pay the full cost of their medication until they pay a total of $310. Some plans have a lower deductible and many have no deductible at all.

Initial Coverage Phase

During the Initial Coverage Phase, Medicare Part D members pay co-pays for their medications based on the tier to which the medication is assigned in the formulary.

In 2014, the Initial Coverage Phase lasts from after the annual deductible has been met until $2,850 worth of medications have been used. It is important to note the $2,850 is a actual value of the medications - not the amount of co-pays paid by the member.

As an example, if the medication has a retail price of $160 but the member pays a co-pay of $40 based on it being a Tier 3 medication in the plan's formulary, the amount that counts toward the $2,850 threshold is $160.

Coverage Gap - Or "Donut Hole"

After the threshold of $2,850 has been reached, the member enters into phase known as the Coverage Gap. This phase is also commonly known as the "Donut Hole."

Fortunately, the Coverage Gap is not now as penal as it has been in the past.

In earlier years, members would pay 100 percent of the retail cost of their medications during the Coverage Gap. In the aforementioned example, the member would go from paying $40 in the Initial Coverage Phase to $160 in the Coverage Gap.

In 2013, a member will pay 47.5 percent of the retail cost of the medication during the Coverage Gap. Therefore, instead of paying the $160 in the example, the member would pay 47.5 percent of $160 - or $76.

Catastrophic Phase

After the member spends $4,550 in True Out-of-Pocket costs (TROOP) on medications, he or she will enter into the Catastrophic Phase in which their costs will decrease dramatically.

In the Catastrophic Phase, members pay the greater of 5 percent of the retail cost of their medication or $2.65 for generics and $6.60 for brand-name medications.

Importantly, the calculation of the $4,550 TROOP is not the actual cost the member spends. Instead, the member receives credit for 100 percent of the retail price of medications purchased while in the Coverage Gap though the member only actually paid 47.5 percent of the retail price.

Because of this additional credit given to the member, the actual money spent by the member prior to reaching the Catastrophic Phase is significantly less than $4,550.

In fact, for a plan with no deductible, the actual amount spent prior to reaching the Catastrophic Phase is likely between $2,600 and $2,800. For a plan with a deductible of $325, the actual amount spent is likely between $2,750 and $2,950.

Though the estimated out-of-pocket cost is higher for plans with a deductible, this difference is usually more than offset by the lower monthly premium for the plan with the deductible. Monthly premiums do not count toward the TROOP calculation.

Ways To Minimize Drug Costs

There are three key strategies a Medicare beneficiary can use to minimize the amount spent every year on prescription medications.

www.medicare.gov

The Center for Medicare and Medicaid Services (CMS) - the government department that administers Medicare - offers a website that provides a tremendous amount of information for Medicare beneficiaries.

This website - www.medicare.gov - includes an online tool through which Medicare beneficiaries can input their medications and dosages and the website will produce a report showing the Medicare Part D drug plan that will cost the least for them. This report includes all total costs including monthly premiums, deductibles and co-pays as well as costs through all coverage phases.

The website also allows the Medicare beneficiary to review the CMS quality ratings for plans as well as enroll online.

If the Medicare beneficiary is interested in a Medicare Advantage plan, he or she can also receive a report showing their estimated drug costs under the Medicare Part D drug plans included with the Medicare Advantage plans offered in their area.

Use of Generic Medications

More and more brand name medications are becoming generic due to the expiration of the patents held by the pharmaceutical companies that originally developed them. This includes popular medications such as Lipitor (Atorvastatin), Plavix (Clopidogrel) and Singulair (Montelukast).

A Medicare beneficiary should migrate to a generic any time the opportunity exists. This includes not just switching from a brand to its generic but also, if appropriate and working closely with their doctor, evaluating switching from a brand to a generic of the same medication class even if the generic does not have identical active ingredients.

Most Medicare Part D plans will actively encourage their members to migrate to generic medications when possible as a way of bringing down the overall cost for everyone.

Having said this, it is not always possible to switch to a generic of the same medication class due to such individual considerations as interactions with other medications, allergies as well as past history which may have shown a brand medication to work better than a generic substitute.

Delaying or Avoiding the Coverage Gap

When a Medicare beneficiary uses medications that subjects him or her to entering the Coverage Gap (Donut Hole), an effective strategy to reducing costs can be to obtain generics without using his or her Medicare Part D coverage.

Pharmacies such as Wal-Mart, Walgreens and Target offer many of the same generic medications used by Medicare beneficiaries with co-pays comparable or even lower than required under the member's Medicare Part D plan.

However, if the member gets generics from a pharmacy such as Wal-Mart and does not provide his or her Medicare Part D card, these generics will not count toward the annual Coverage Gap calculation.

This can help the member delay or sometimes even avoid reaching the Coverage Gap at which time medication costs increase.

Importantly, because pharmacies will keep a customer's insurance information in their computer system, it is a good idea to use two separate pharmacies when emplying this strategy. Use one pharmacy for medication in which the member uses his or her Medicare Part D coverage and another pharmacy such as Wal-Mart or Target for generics not using the Medicare Part D coverage.

Medicare Enrollment Periods

There are specific times during which a Medicare beneficiary can enroll in a Medicare plan or change their plan.

Medicare Part A

Providing the potential Medicare beneficiary or their qualifying spouse has met the minimum requirements for contributing to the Medicare system through Medicare payroll taxes during their working career, a person becomes eligible for Medicare Part A the first day of the month in which they turn 65 years old.

For example, a person born on September 15, 1949 will be eligible for Medicare Part A beginning September 1, 2014.

Interestingly, if someone's birthday falls on the 1st day of the month, their Medicare Part A will begin on the 1st day of the previous month. As an example, a person who was born on November 1, 1949 will be eligible for Medicare Part A on October 1, 2014.

Generally, CMS will send a new Medicare beneficiary their Medicare card showing their effective dates around 3.5 months prior to their Medicare Part A effective date.

Medicare Part B - Turning 65

The effective date for Medicare Part B is a little more complicated than Part A.

The Social Security Administration (SSA) manages enrollment in Medicare Part B. When an imminent Medicare beneficiary approaches their Medicare Part A effective date - the first day of the month in which they turn 65 years old - SSA makes an assumption about whether the beneficiary wishes to have their Medicare Part B take effect based on whether they have begun to collect Social Security.

If the imminent Medicare beneficiary has begun to collect Social Security by the 65th birthday, SSA assumes they wish to have their Medicare Part B take effect. Accordingly, when CMS sends the new Medicare beneficiary their new Medicare card, it will show an effective date for Medicare Part B as the same effective date for Medicare Part A.

However, if the new Medicare beneficiary is not collecting Social Security benefits by the time they reach age 65, SSA assumes they do not wish to have Medicare Part B take effect at the same time as Medicare Part A. The reason for this is SSA assumes the new Medicare beneficiary is still working and is receiving health insurance through their employer.

Importantly, this assumption is not correct for many new Medicare beneficiaries.

Many new Medicare beneficiaries want or need to have their Medicare Part B take effect at the same time as their Medicare Part A but are delaying the start of their Social Security benefits.

Conversely, many new Medicare beneficiaries have started to collect Social Security benefits but have alternative health coverage through their or their spouse's employer and do not need Medicare Part B to take effect at the same time as they become eligible for Medicare Part A.

A Medicare beneficiary who is not automatically enrolled in Medicare Part B due to not yet collecting Social Security benefits will need to enroll either by going online at www.socialsecurity.gov, calling Social Security at (800) 772-1213 or by visiting their local Social Security office.

While it may not be the most convenient, visiting the local Social Security can eliminate some snags sometime experienced with on-line or telephonic enrollment. It is recommended to call ahead and make and appointment. Also, the first and the last days of the month tend to be more crowded at the Social Security office than other days.

Medicare Part B - Special Enrollment Periods

If a Medicare beneficiary does not elect Medicare Part B when they are first eligible because they still have health coverage from an employer, they will be allowed to enroll using a Special Election Period (SEP) when they lose or disenroll from such employer coverage. In most situations, such Medicare beneficiaries can leave employee coverage at any time and choose to enroll in Medicare Part B.

If a Medicare beneficiary does not elect Medicare Part B when first eligible but does not have other credible coverage, they can enroll in Medicare Part B in the future only during specific times of the year. These times are between January and March of each year for Medicare Part B coverage that will take effect the following July 1.

Medicare may assess a Medicare Part B Late-Enrollment Penalty in a situation where a Medicare member did not have credible alternative coverage when first eligible for Medicare Part B.

Medicare Supplements

Most Medicare Supplement carriers allow a new Medicare beneficiary to enroll up to 6 months prior to their Medicare Part B effective date. Obviously, the coverage does not become active until both Medicare Part A and Medicare Part B are effective. Most carriers require the first month's premium be collected at the time of enrollment.

It is important to note, since most Medicare beneficiaries who choose a Medicare Supplement will also need a stand-alone Medicare Part D plan, CMS does not allow new Medicare beneficiaries to enroll in a Medicare Part D plan until they are within 3 months of their Medicare Part A effective date.

Medicare Advantage and Medicare Part D - Turning 65

Medicare beneficiaries who elect Medicare Part B when they are first eligible have a 7-month window to enroll in a Medicare Advantage or Medicare Part D drug plan. This 7-month window includes the three months prior to the month in which they turn 65 and go on Medicare Part B, the actual month they turn 65 and go on Medicare Part B and the three months after they turn 65 and go on Medicare Part B.

Medicare Advantage and Medicare Part D - Annual Enrollment Period

Medicare Beneficiaries can either enroll in, disenroll from or change a Medicare Advantage or Medicare Part D drug plan during the Annual Enrollment Period. For 2014, the Annual Enrollment Period begins on October 15 and lasts until December 7.

Medicare Advantage and Medicare Part D - Special Election Period

There are several situations that provide a Medicare beneficiary a chance to make a change in his or her Medicare Advantage or Medicare Part D coverage outside of the Turning 65 or Annual Enrollment Period. These Special Election Periods (SEPs) include:

- Someone who receives extra financial help to pay for either prescriptions, premiums or co-pays due to low income

- Someone who moves from one county to another

- Someone who disenrolls from other health insurance such as employer's insurance

Extra Assistance

States provide extra assistance for Medicare beneficiaries who have incomes below certain thresholds.

In 2014 those thresholds and the qualifying assistance are as follows:

Monthly Income Single/Married	Benefit	Assistance
$1,458/$1,966	Low Income Subsidy (LIS)	Pay only $2.55 or $6.35 for Part D medications
$1,187/$1,593	Specified Low-Income Medicare Beneficiary (SLMB)	LIS benefits plus State pays $104.90 monthly Medicare Part B Premium
$993/$1,331	Qualified Medicare Beneficiary (QMB)	LIS and SLMB benefits plus State pays co-pays, coinsurance and deductibles

There are also additional asset limitations that must not be exceeded to qualify for extra assistance.

Someone who believes they may qualify for extra assistance should contact their state Medicaid office or can start by calling 1-800-MEDICARE.

Working With an Insurance Agent

Medicare insurance agents can provide a tremendous amount of assistance both in understanding and selecting Medicare plan options as well as continuing to evaluate Medicare options going forward.

However, Medicare insurance agents are only useful if they are compensated based on what is best for the Medicare beneficiary rather than what is best for the insurance carrier that is paying them.

Captive Agents

Captive agents are insurance agents who only represent one insurance carrier and often only one plan. These are often newly-licensed agents who have been selling Medicare insurance less than a year or two and are hired to sell a specific plan rather than assist the Medicare beneficiary in choosing the best plan for their needs.

A captive agent will often have a conflict between the plan that is best for the Medicare beneficiary and a different plan that is the only one he or she is able to sell.

It is not in the best interest of any Medicare beneficiary to rely on a captive agent to assist them in selecting a Medicare insurance plan.

Independent Agents

Unlike captive agents, independent agents usually do represent many different plan types and carriers and are in a position to assist a Medicare beneficiary is selecting the best plan for their needs. Even with an independent agent, it is a good idea for the Medicare beneficiary to ask the agent both what plan types and carriers they represent as well as which ones they do not represent.

If there is a plan type or carrier they do not represent, the Medicare beneficiary may not learn about the plan type or carrier that best meets his or her needs.

A Medicare beneficiary can always call SeniorAssured Insurance at (800) 385-9160 or visit www.seniorassured.com to talk with an independent agent who represents all plan types and major carriers.

About The Author

Charles Bradshaw assists people who are going on Medicare or who are already on Medicare in choosing the right Medicare plan for their needs and budget.

After graduating from the University of Tennessee, Charles worked around the country in Finance, Marketing and executive-level positions helping such companies as Disney, Nestle, Procter and Gamble, DirecTv and Hilton Hotels. He spent enough time doing this work to realize that there was a lot more important decisions affecting people's lives made by real people around kitchen tables than phony people around boardroom tables.

Charles has met with and helped thousands of seniors understand their Medicare options and helped them choose the right plan for their needs. Besides helping people with their Medicare and making a difference in their lives, he considers his greatest professional accomplishment to not having been bitten by any of his clients' dogs though he once was pecked by one of their chickens.

Charles Bradshaw is the Founder and President of MyMedicareAnswer.com.

He can be reached at (800) 385-9160 or via email at **chbradshaw@gmail.com**.

You can also visit MyMedicareAsnwer.com at **www.mymedicareanswer.com**.

www.ingramcontent.com/pod-product-compliance
Lightning Source LLC
Chambersburg PA
CBHW030535290526
45786CB00004B/1725